I0710158

Notes / Ex

Table of contents

Chapter 1: Understanding the Love Language of Dogs

The Importance of Understanding Your Dog's Needs

Understanding your dog's needs is crucial in building a strong and loving relationship with your furry companion. Dogs, like humans, have basic needs that must be met in order for them to thrive both physically and emotionally. By understanding and fulfilling these needs, you can ensure that your dog is happy, healthy, and well-adjusted.

One of the most important needs of a dog is exercise. Dogs are active creatures by nature and require regular physical activity to maintain their overall health and well-being. By incorporating daily walks, playtime, and other forms of exercise into your dog's routine, you can help them stay fit, mentally stimulated, and prevent behavioral issues that may arise from pent-up energy.

Another crucial need for dogs is a safe and comfortable environment. Providing your dog with a cozy bed, access to fresh water, nutritious food, and a secure space to call their own is essential in creating a sense of security and belonging. Dogs thrive in environments where they feel safe and loved, so it's important to make sure their living space is clean, organized, and free from hazards.

In addition to physical needs, dogs also have emotional needs that must be met in order for them to feel loved and secure. Dogs are social animals and crave companionship, attention, and affection from their human family members. By spending quality time with your dog, engaging in bonding activities, and showing them love and affection, you can strengthen your relationship and create a deep and lasting bond.

By taking the time to understand and meet your dog's needs, you can ensure that they live a happy, healthy, and fulfilling life. Whether you are a seasoned dog owner or a prospective pet parent, it's important to prioritize your dog's well-being and make their needs a top priority. By doing so, you can create a loving and harmonious relationship with your furry friend that will last a lifetime.

Building Trust and Connection with Your Dog

Building trust and connection with your dog is essential for a happy and healthy relationship. Whether you have a new puppy or a senior dog, it's important to establish a strong bond based on trust and love. By following some simple tips and techniques, you can strengthen your relationship with your furry friend and create a deep and lasting connection.

One of the best ways to build trust with your dog is through positive reinforcement training. Rewarding good behavior with treats, praise, and affection will help your dog associate you with positive experiences. Consistency is key when it comes to training, so make sure to set clear boundaries and stick to them. By using positive reinforcement techniques, you can build a strong foundation of trust and communication with your dog.

Another important aspect of building trust with your dog is to create a safe and comfortable environment for them. Make sure your dog has a cozy bed, plenty of toys, and access to fresh water and food. Providing a safe and secure space for your dog will help them feel relaxed and at ease, which will strengthen your bond.

Incorporating exercise and play into your dog's routine is another great way to build trust and connection. Taking your dog for daily walks, playing fetch in the backyard, or engaging in interactive games will not only provide physical exercise but also mental stimulation. A tired and happy dog is more likely to trust and bond with you, so make sure to incorporate plenty of playtime into your daily routine.

Overall, building trust and connection with your dog takes time, patience, and dedication. By using positive reinforcement training, creating a safe environment, and incorporating exercise and play into your dog's routine, you can strengthen your bond and create a loving and lasting relationship with your furry friend. Remember to communicate effectively, show love and care, and celebrate special occasions with your dog to further enhance your connection.

Recognizing Signs of Affection from Your Dog

As dog owners, one of the most rewarding aspects of having a canine companion is the love and affection they show us. Dogs have a unique way of expressing their feelings, and it's important for us to recognize the signs of affection they display. By understanding these cues, we can deepen our bond with our furry friends and ensure they feel loved and cared for.

One common sign of affection from your dog is wagging their tail. While many people believe that a wagging tail automatically means a dog is happy, it's important to pay attention to the way your dog is wagging their tail. A loose, relaxed wag usually indicates a happy and content pup, while a stiff or rapid wag could signal excitement or even aggression. Tail wagging is just one way dogs communicate their emotions, so be sure to consider other body language cues as well.

Another telltale sign of affection from your dog is cuddling. Whether your dog likes to snuggle up next to you on the couch or rest their head on your lap, physical closeness is a clear sign of trust and affection. Dogs are pack animals by nature, so seeking out physical contact with their human family members is a way for them to feel safe and secure. Embrace these moments of closeness and enjoy the warmth and companionship your dog provides.

In addition to tail wagging and cuddling, your dog may also show affection through licking. While some people may find this behavior off-putting, licking is a natural way for dogs to show love and affection. Dogs groom each other as a way of bonding, and when your dog licks you, they are essentially "grooming" you as a sign of their attachment. If you find excessive licking bothersome, you can redirect this behavior by offering your dog a toy or treat to chew on instead.

Lastly, pay attention to your dog's facial expressions. Just like humans, dogs have a wide range of facial expressions that convey their emotions. A relaxed, open mouth with a slightly lolling tongue is a sign of contentment, while narrowed eyes or a tense jaw could indicate stress or discomfort. By observing your dog's facial expressions and overall body language, you can better understand their emotional state and respond accordingly to show them love and support.

In conclusion, recognizing the signs of affection from your dog is essential for strengthening your bond and ensuring a happy, healthy relationship. Whether it's through tail wagging, cuddling, licking, or facial expressions, your dog has unique ways of showing you how much they care. By paying attention to these cues and responding with love and affection of your own, you can create a deep and meaningful connection with your canine companion that will last a lifetime.

Chapter 2: Bonding with Your Dog Through Training

Positive Reinforcement Training Techniques

Positive reinforcement training techniques are a powerful tool for dog owners looking to build a strong and loving bond with their furry companions. By using positive reinforcement, you can encourage good behavior in your dog while fostering a relationship built on trust and respect. This approach focuses on rewarding desired behaviors with treats, praise, or playtime, rather than punishing undesirable actions. By consistently using positive reinforcement, you can effectively communicate with your dog and strengthen your connection.

One of the key principles of positive reinforcement training is to reward your dog immediately after they exhibit the desired behavior. This instant feedback helps your dog understand what they did right and encourages them to repeat the behavior in the future. When your dog knows that good behavior leads to positive outcomes, they are more likely to engage in those behaviors consistently. By using treats, toys, or verbal praise as rewards, you can show your dog love and appreciation for their efforts.

Consistency is crucial when it comes to positive reinforcement training. It's important to set clear expectations for your dog and stick to them consistently. By providing consistent feedback and rewards, you can help your dog understand what is expected of them and reinforce good behavior over time. Consistency also helps build trust between you and your dog, as they learn to rely on you for guidance and support.

Incorporating play and exercise into your dog's routine is another important aspect of positive reinforcement training. By engaging in fun and interactive activities with your dog, you can strengthen your bond and provide mental and physical stimulation. Playtime can also be used as a reward for good behavior, making training sessions more enjoyable for both you and your dog. By incorporating play and exercise into your daily routine, you can show your dog love and care in a way that promotes their overall well-being.

Overall, positive reinforcement training techniques are a valuable tool for dog owners looking to build a loving and respectful relationship with their pets. By using rewards, praise, and play as motivators, you can encourage good behavior in your dog and strengthen your bond over time. Consistency, clear communication, and incorporating play and exercise into your routine are key components of successful positive reinforcement training. By implementing these techniques, you can show love and care to your dog while fostering a strong and lasting relationship based on trust and mutual respect.

Establishing a Routine for Training and Play

Establishing a routine for training and play is essential for building a strong bond with your furry friend. Consistency is key when it comes to teaching your dog new tricks or behaviors. By setting aside dedicated time each day for training sessions, you can help your dog understand what is expected of them and reinforce positive behaviors. Incorporating playtime into your routine is also important for keeping your dog mentally and physically stimulated.

Training your dog not only helps them learn new skills, but it also strengthens the bond between you and your furry companion. Positive reinforcement techniques, such as using treats or praise, can be highly effective in encouraging good behavior. It's important to be patient and understanding during training sessions, as every dog learns at their own pace. By being consistent and using positive reinforcement, you can help your dog feel loved and secure.

For senior dogs, training and play may look a bit different than for younger pups. It's important to take your dog's age and physical limitations into account when establishing a routine. Gentle exercises and mental stimulation can help keep your senior dog feeling young at heart. By showing them love and patience during training sessions, you can help them maintain their cognitive abilities and physical health.

Rescue dogs often come with their own set of challenges, but with patience and love, they can thrive in their new home. Establishing a routine for training and play is crucial for helping rescue dogs adjust to their new environment and build trust with their new family. By showing them love and understanding, you can help your rescue dog feel safe and secure in their new home.

Overall, incorporating training and play into your dog's routine is essential for building a strong and loving bond with your furry friend. Whether you have a senior dog, a rescue dog, or a puppy, taking the time to train and play with them shows them that they are loved and valued members of your family. By being patient, consistent, and understanding, you can create a positive and enriching environment for your dog to thrive in.

Building Confidence in Your Dog Through Training

Training your dog is not only about teaching them basic commands and behaviors, but it is also an opportunity to build their confidence. When a dog is confident, they are more likely to feel secure in their environment and have a positive outlook on life. By incorporating training into your daily routine, you can help your dog develop the skills and self-assurance they need to thrive.

One of the key ways to build confidence in your dog through training is to set them up for success. Start with simple commands and gradually increase the difficulty as your dog becomes more comfortable and confident. Use positive reinforcement techniques, such as treats and praise, to reward your dog for good behavior and encourage them to continue learning and growing.

Consistency is also crucial when it comes to training your dog and building their confidence. Set aside dedicated time each day to work on training exercises with your dog, and be patient and understanding as they learn. Remember that every dog is unique and will progress at their own pace, so it is important to be supportive and encouraging throughout the training process.

Incorporating play and exercise into your dog's routine can also help boost their confidence. Engaging in activities such as fetch, agility training, or interactive games can help your dog build physical and mental strength, as well as improve their overall well-being. These activities can also strengthen the bond between you and your dog, which is essential for building trust and confidence.

As a dog owner, it is important to remember that building confidence in your dog through training is a lifelong journey. By continuing to work with your dog on a regular basis and providing them with the love and support they need, you can help them become the confident and happy companion you both deserve. Together, you can conquer challenges and celebrate successes, creating a strong and trusting relationship that will last a lifetime.

Chapter 3: Showing Love to Your Senior Dog

Understanding the Needs of Aging Dogs

As our furry companions age, their needs and behaviors may change, requiring us to adapt our care and attention to ensure they continue to live happy and healthy lives. Understanding the needs of aging dogs is essential for providing them with the proper care and support they require in their later years. By recognizing and addressing these needs, we can help our senior dogs maintain their quality of life and enjoy their golden years to the fullest.

One of the most important aspects of caring for an aging dog is monitoring their health and well-being. As dogs get older, they may develop age-related health issues such as arthritis, dental problems, or vision and hearing loss. Regular veterinary check-ups and screenings can help identify and address these issues early on, allowing for timely treatment and management. It is also crucial to provide a nutritious diet tailored to their specific needs, as well as regular exercise to keep them active and maintain their muscle tone and mobility.

In addition to physical health, it is essential to consider the emotional and mental well-being of aging dogs. As they age, dogs may experience changes in their behavior, such as increased anxiety, confusion, or aggression. Providing a safe and comfortable environment, along with plenty of love and attention, can help alleviate these issues and make them feel secure and loved. Bonding with your aging dog through training and positive reinforcement can also strengthen your relationship and provide mental stimulation, keeping their minds sharp and engaged.

For families with aging dogs, it is important to involve everyone in the care and attention of their senior companion. Educating children about the needs of aging dogs and how to interact with them respectfully and gently can help create a harmonious and loving environment for the entire family. By incorporating exercise and play into your dog's routine, you can keep them active and engaged, promoting physical and mental well-being while strengthening the bond between you and your furry friend.

In conclusion, understanding the needs of aging dogs is crucial for providing them with the love, care, and support they require in their later years. By monitoring their health, providing a nutritious diet, and creating a safe and loving environment, we can help our senior dogs live happy and fulfilling lives. Through bonding, training, and regular exercise, we can strengthen our relationship with them and ensure they feel loved and cherished every day. By celebrating special occasions and creating lasting memories with our aging dogs, we can show them how much they mean to us and make the most of the time we have together.

Providing Comfort and Support for Senior Dogs

As our beloved canine companions age, they may require extra comfort and support to ensure they live out their golden years in peace and contentment. Providing comfort and support for senior dogs is essential in helping them maintain their quality of life and feel loved and cared for. In this subchapter, we will explore various ways in which you can provide comfort and support for your senior dog, ensuring they feel safe, secure, and cherished.

One of the most important ways to provide comfort for senior dogs is by creating a safe and comfortable environment for them to live in. This may involve making adjustments to your home, such as adding ramps or stairs to help them navigate around the house more easily, providing a soft and cozy bed for them to rest in, or ensuring they have easy access to food, water, and a bathroom area. By creating a comfortable environment for your senior dog, you can help them feel secure and at ease in their surroundings.

Another way to provide comfort and support for senior dogs is by ensuring they receive proper medical care and attention. As dogs age, they may develop health issues that require special treatment or medication. It is important to work closely with your veterinarian to address any health concerns your senior dog may have and to ensure they receive the care they need to stay healthy and comfortable. Regular check-ups, vaccinations, and screenings can help catch any potential health problems early and ensure your senior dog receives the proper treatment.

In addition to medical care, providing comfort and support for senior dogs also involves meeting their emotional and social needs. Senior dogs may experience loneliness, anxiety, or depression as they age, especially if they are dealing with health issues or the loss of a companion. Spending quality time with your senior dog, giving them plenty of attention, and engaging in activities they enjoy can help alleviate feelings of loneliness and provide them with comfort and companionship. Additionally, socializing your senior dog with other dogs or people can help keep them mentally stimulated and emotionally fulfilled.

As your senior dog continues to age, their dietary needs may change, requiring you to adjust their diet to meet their changing nutritional requirements. Providing a balanced and nutritious diet tailored to your senior dog's specific needs can help support their overall health and well-being. Consult with your veterinarian to determine the best diet for your senior dog and make any necessary adjustments to ensure they receive the proper nutrients to keep them healthy and comfortable.

In conclusion, providing comfort and support for senior dogs is essential in helping them live out their twilight years with love, dignity, and compassion. By creating a safe and comfortable environment, ensuring they receive proper medical care, meeting their emotional and social needs, and adjusting their diet as necessary, you can help your senior dog feel cherished and cared for as they age. Your senior dog has given you a lifetime of love and companionship – now it's your turn to show them the same level of care and devotion in return.

Adjusting Your Routine to Accommodate Senior Dogs

As our dogs age, it's important for us as pet owners to adjust our routines to accommodate their changing needs. Senior dogs may not be as active or energetic as they once were, and it's our responsibility to ensure they are comfortable and happy in their golden years. Making simple adjustments to your daily routine can make a world of difference in your senior dog's quality of life.

One way to adjust your routine for your senior dog is to incorporate more breaks and rest periods throughout the day. Older dogs may not have the stamina they once did, so it's important to give them plenty of opportunities to rest and relax. Consider taking shorter walks or play sessions, and be mindful of signs of fatigue or discomfort in your senior pup.

Another important adjustment to make for senior dogs is to pay closer attention to their dietary needs. As dogs age, their metabolism slows down and they may require a different type of food or portion size to maintain a healthy weight. Consult with your veterinarian to determine the best diet for your senior dog, and consider incorporating supplements or senior-specific dog food to support their aging bodies.

In addition to adjusting their exercise and diet, it's also important to create a safe and comfortable environment for your senior dog. Make sure their bed is soft and supportive, and consider adding ramps or stairs to help them navigate around the house more easily. Keep their living space free of hazards and clutter to prevent accidents or injuries.

Lastly, don't forget to show your senior dog plenty of love and affection. Spend quality time with them, cuddle up on the couch, and shower them with praise and attention. Senior dogs may require a bit more patience and understanding, but the love and loyalty they give in return is truly priceless. Adjusting your routine to accommodate your senior dog is a simple yet meaningful way to show them how much you care.

Chapter 4: Loving and Caring for Your Rescue Dog

Building Trust with a Rescue Dog

Rescue dogs often come with a history of neglect or trauma, which can make it challenging to build trust with them. However, with patience, love, and understanding, you can create a strong bond with your rescue dog. One of the first steps in building trust with a rescue dog is giving them space and time to adjust to their new environment. Allow them to explore their surroundings at their own pace and avoid overwhelming them with too much attention or affection too soon.

Consistency is key when building trust with a rescue dog. Establish a routine for feeding, walking, and playtime, so your dog knows what to expect. This will help them feel safe and secure in their new home. Positive reinforcement training is also essential in building trust with a rescue dog. Use treats, praise, and gentle guidance to reward good behavior and show your dog that you are a trustworthy and loving caregiver.

Creating a safe and comfortable environment for your rescue dog is crucial in building trust. Provide them with a cozy bed, toys, and a designated space where they can retreat when they feel overwhelmed. Make sure your home is free of any hazards that could cause anxiety or stress for your dog. Additionally, be patient and understanding with your rescue dog. Building trust takes time, and it's important to be patient and consistent in your efforts to create a strong bond with your new furry friend.

Another way to build trust with a rescue dog is to incorporate exercise and play into their routine. Regular physical activity not only helps keep your dog healthy but also strengthens the bond between you. Take your dog for walks, play fetch in the backyard, or engage in interactive games that stimulate their mind and body. This will help your rescue dog feel happy, loved, and secure in their new home.

Overall, building trust with a rescue dog requires patience, love, and dedication. By providing a safe and comfortable environment, establishing a routine, using positive reinforcement training, and incorporating exercise and play into their routine, you can create a strong bond with your rescue dog. Remember that every dog is unique, and it may take time for your rescue dog to fully trust you. But with time, patience, and love, you can build a lasting and meaningful relationship with your new furry companion.

Addressing Behavioral Issues in Rescue Dogs

Rescue dogs often come with a history that may include neglect, abuse, or trauma, which can manifest in behavioral issues. It is important for dog owners to understand and address these issues with patience, compassion, and proper training. One common behavioral issue in rescue dogs is separation anxiety, which can lead to destructive behavior when left alone. It is crucial to gradually desensitize the dog to being alone and provide them with a safe and comfortable space to relax in your absence.

Another common behavioral issue in rescue dogs is fear and aggression towards other animals or humans. This can be a result of past experiences or lack of socialization. It is important to work with a professional trainer to help your rescue dog overcome their fears and learn to trust again. Positive reinforcement training, patience, and consistency are key in addressing these behavioral issues.

Some rescue dogs may exhibit resource guarding behavior, where they become possessive over food, toys, or other items. This can be a result of insecurity or a lack of resources in their past. It is important to establish trust with your rescue dog through positive reinforcement training and gradually work on desensitizing them to sharing resources. Providing a structured routine and clear boundaries can also help alleviate resource guarding behavior.

It is important to remember that rescue dogs may take time to adjust to their new environment and build trust with their new family. It is crucial to be patient, understanding, and consistent in your training efforts. Building a strong bond with your rescue dog through positive reinforcement, play, and exercise can help address behavioral issues and strengthen your relationship.

Overall, addressing behavioral issues in rescue dogs requires time, patience, and understanding. By working with a professional trainer, providing a structured routine, and showing love and compassion, you can help your rescue dog overcome their past and thrive in their new home. Remember to celebrate the progress your rescue dog makes and always prioritize their well-being and happiness.

Creating a Safe and Loving Environment for Rescue Dogs

Creating a safe and loving environment for rescue dogs is essential in helping them adjust to their new home and overcome any past traumas they may have experienced. When bringing a rescue dog into your home, it is important to remember that they may be scared, anxious, or unsure of their surroundings. By creating a safe and loving environment, you can help them feel more comfortable and secure.

One of the first steps in creating a safe and loving environment for a rescue dog is to provide them with a designated space that is their own. This could be a cozy crate, a comfortable bed, or a quiet corner of the room where they can retreat to when they need some time alone. By giving them their own space, you are providing them with a sense of security and privacy that can help reduce their anxiety.

Another important aspect of creating a safe and loving environment for rescue dogs is to establish a routine. Dogs thrive on routine and knowing what to expect, so by setting a consistent schedule for feeding, walks, and playtime, you can help them feel more secure in their new environment. This routine can also help build trust and strengthen the bond between you and your rescue dog.

In addition to providing a safe space and establishing a routine, it is important to show your rescue dog love and patience. Many rescue dogs have been through traumatic experiences and may be slow to trust or show affection. By being patient, understanding, and gentle with your rescue dog, you can help them feel safe and loved in their new home.

Overall, creating a safe and loving environment for rescue dogs is essential in helping them adjust to their new surroundings and build trust with their new family. By providing them with a designated space, establishing a routine, and showing them love and patience, you can help your rescue dog feel more comfortable and secure in their new home. Remember, rescue dogs may come with their own set of challenges, but with time, patience, and love, they can thrive and become a beloved member of your family.

Chapter 5: Strengthening the Relationship with Your Anxious Dog

Understanding the Causes of Anxiety in Dogs

Many dog owners may notice that their furry friends experience anxiety from time to time. Understanding the causes of anxiety in dogs can help pet owners provide the necessary support and care for their beloved companions. There are several factors that can contribute to anxiety in dogs, including genetics, past experiences, lack of socialization, changes in environment, and medical conditions.

Genetics play a significant role in a dog's predisposition to anxiety. Certain breeds are more prone to anxiety than others, such as German Shepherds, Border Collies, and Cocker Spaniels. If a dog comes from a line of anxious parents, they may be more likely to develop anxiety themselves. It is essential for prospective dog owners to research breeds and their typical behaviors to better understand what to expect in terms of anxiety levels.

Past experiences can also contribute to anxiety in dogs. Dogs that have been neglected, abused, or abandoned may develop anxiety as a result of their traumatic experiences. It is crucial for pet owners to provide a loving and stable environment for their dogs to help them overcome past traumas and build trust and confidence.

Lack of socialization can lead to anxiety in dogs. Dogs that have not been exposed to a variety of people, animals, and environments may feel overwhelmed and anxious in new situations. It is important for pet owners to socialize their dogs from a young age to help them feel more comfortable and confident in different settings.

Changes in environment can trigger anxiety in dogs. Moving to a new home, introducing a new pet or family member, or even rearranging furniture can disrupt a dog's sense of security and cause anxiety. It is essential for pet owners to provide a stable and consistent environment for their dogs to help them feel safe and secure.

Medical conditions, such as thyroid disorders, epilepsy, or arthritis, can also contribute to anxiety in dogs. It is important for pet owners to monitor their dog's health and seek veterinary care if they suspect their dog is experiencing anxiety as a result of an underlying medical condition. By understanding the causes of anxiety in dogs, pet owners can provide the necessary support and care to help their furry friends feel safe, secure, and loved.

Creating a Calm and Secure Environment for Anxious Dogs

Creating a calm and secure environment for anxious dogs is crucial in helping them feel safe and comfortable in their surroundings. Anxious dogs can exhibit a wide range of behaviors, from excessive barking and whining to destructive chewing and aggression. By creating a safe and secure environment, you can help your anxious dog feel more at ease and reduce their stress levels.

One way to create a calm and secure environment for anxious dogs is to establish a consistent routine. Dogs thrive on routine and knowing what to expect, so try to feed them, walk them, and play with them at the same times each day. This will help your dog feel more secure and reduce their anxiety levels.

Another way to create a calm and secure environment for anxious dogs is to provide them with a safe space where they can retreat when they feel overwhelmed. This could be a crate, a cozy bed, or a quiet corner of the house where they can relax and unwind. Make sure this space is always available to your dog and never use it as a form of punishment.

In addition to establishing a routine and providing a safe space, it's important to create a calm and peaceful atmosphere in your home. Avoid loud noises, sudden movements, and chaotic environments that can trigger anxiety in your dog. Instead, try to create a soothing environment with soft lighting, calming music, and comfortable bedding.

By creating a calm and secure environment for your anxious dog, you can help them feel more at ease and reduce their stress levels. Remember to be patient and understanding with your anxious dog, as it may take time for them to adjust to their new environment. With love, patience, and consistency, you can help your anxious dog feel safe and secure in their home.

Implementing Techniques to Help Anxious Dogs Overcome Their Fears

Implementing techniques to help anxious dogs overcome their fears can greatly improve their quality of life and strengthen the bond between you and your furry companion. Dogs, like humans, can experience anxiety for various reasons such as past trauma, lack of socialization, or genetic predisposition. As responsible pet owners, it is our duty to help our anxious dogs feel safe and secure in their environment.

One effective technique to help anxious dogs is desensitization. This involves exposing your dog to the source of their fear in a controlled and gradual manner. For example, if your dog is afraid of loud noises, you can start by playing recordings of the noises at a low volume and gradually increase the volume over time. This gradual exposure can help your dog become more comfortable and less fearful of the trigger.

Another technique that can be effective in helping anxious dogs is counterconditioning. This involves pairing the source of your dog's fear with something positive, such as treats or toys. For example, if your dog is afraid of strangers, you can have strangers give your dog treats or play with them to create positive associations. Over time, your dog may come to see strangers as a source of positive experiences rather than fear.

It is important to create a safe and comfortable environment for your anxious dog. This may involve providing a quiet and secure space for them to retreat to when they are feeling overwhelmed. You can also use calming aids such as pheromone diffusers or calming music to help reduce their anxiety. Consistency and patience are key when implementing these techniques, as it may take time for your anxious dog to overcome their fears.

By implementing these techniques and showing patience and understanding, you can help your anxious dog feel more secure and confident in their environment. Remember that every dog is unique, and what works for one dog may not work for another. It is important to consult with a professional trainer or behaviorist if your dog's anxiety is severe or persistent. With love, patience, and the right techniques, you can help your anxious dog overcome their fears and live a happy and fulfilling life.

Chapter 6: Incorporating Exercise and Play into Your Dog's Routine

The Benefits of Regular Exercise for Dogs

Regular exercise is crucial for the overall health and well-being of our canine companions. Just like humans, dogs need physical activity to maintain a healthy weight, build muscle strength, and keep their minds sharp. One of the benefits of regular exercise for dogs is that it helps prevent obesity, which can lead to a myriad of health issues such as diabetes, heart disease, and joint problems. By incorporating exercise into your dog's routine, you can help them stay fit and healthy for years to come.

In addition to physical health benefits, regular exercise also has a positive impact on a dog's mental well-being. Dogs are naturally active animals, and they need an outlet for their energy to prevent boredom and destructive behaviors. By providing them with regular exercise, you can help reduce their stress and anxiety levels, improve their mood, and strengthen the bond between you and your furry friend. Whether it's going for a walk, playing fetch, or engaging in agility training, regular exercise can help keep your dog happy and content.

Another benefit of regular exercise for dogs is that it can improve their socialization skills. When dogs engage in physical activities such as going to the dog park or attending obedience classes, they have the opportunity to interact with other dogs and people. This can help them develop better social skills, learn how to communicate effectively with other animals, and become more confident in new situations. Regular exercise can also help reduce behavioral issues such as aggression, fearfulness, and separation anxiety, making it easier for your dog to adapt to different environments and situations.

For families with multiple dogs, regular exercise can help strengthen the bond between the animals in the household. When dogs engage in physical activities together, they learn how to work as a team, communicate effectively, and build trust with one another. This can help reduce conflicts and tension between dogs, improve their overall relationship, and create a harmonious living environment for everyone in the family. By making exercise a priority for all of your dogs, you can help them build strong bonds and friendships that will last a lifetime.

Overall, regular exercise is essential for the health and well-being of our canine companions. By incorporating physical activities into your dog's routine, you can help them stay fit, mentally stimulated, and socially engaged. Whether it's going for a run, playing games, or attending training classes, there are countless ways to keep your dog active and happy. So grab a leash, lace up your shoes, and get ready to enjoy the many benefits of regular exercise for your beloved furry friend.

Fun and Engaging Ways to Keep Your Dog Active

Keeping your dog active is not only important for their physical health, but also for their mental well-being. Dogs are naturally active animals, and they need plenty of exercise and mental stimulation to stay happy and healthy. In this subchapter, we will explore fun and engaging ways to keep your dog active, whether you have a young and energetic pup or a senior dog who needs a gentler approach to exercise.

One of the easiest ways to keep your dog active is by taking them for regular walks. Dogs love to explore their surroundings, and going for a walk is a great way for them to burn off excess energy and stay mentally stimulated. Try to vary your walking route to keep things interesting for your dog, and consider incorporating some training exercises into your walk to keep their mind engaged.

Another fun way to keep your dog active is by playing games with them. Dogs love to play, and games like fetch, tug-of-war, and hide-and-seek are great ways to keep them moving and engaged. You can also try setting up an agility course in your backyard or local park for some extra fun and exercise.

If you have a water-loving dog, swimming is a fantastic way to keep them active. Swimming is a low-impact exercise that is easy on your dog's joints, making it ideal for senior dogs or those with mobility issues. Just be sure to supervise your dog closely while they are in the water to ensure their safety.

To keep your dog mentally stimulated, consider incorporating puzzle toys and interactive feeding devices into their routine. These toys require your dog to use their problem-solving skills to access their food or treats, providing them with mental exercise and preventing boredom. You can also try teaching your dog new tricks or commands to keep their mind sharp and engaged.

Overall, the key to keeping your dog active is to find activities that they enjoy and that suit their age, fitness level, and personality. By incorporating a variety of fun and engaging activities into your dog's routine, you can help them stay happy, healthy, and mentally stimulated for years to come. So get out there and have fun with your furry friend!

Creating a Playful Bond with Your Dog Through Interactive Games

Creating a playful bond with your dog through interactive games is a fun and rewarding way to strengthen your relationship with your furry friend. Dogs are naturally playful creatures, and engaging in interactive games with them can provide mental stimulation, physical exercise, and a sense of connection between you and your dog. By incorporating games into your daily routine, you can not only enhance your dog's overall well-being but also create lasting memories together.

Interactive games such as fetch, hide-and-seek, tug-of-war, and puzzle toys are great ways to keep your dog entertained and engaged. These games help to channel your dog's energy in a positive way, prevent boredom, and provide an outlet for their natural instincts. By playing these games with your dog, you are not only providing them with physical exercise but also mental stimulation, which is essential for their overall health and happiness.

Playing interactive games with your dog also helps to build trust and strengthen the bond between you and your furry companion. When you engage in play with your dog, you are creating a positive and enjoyable experience that strengthens your relationship and deepens your connection. Your dog will learn to trust and rely on you as their playmate, which can lead to a stronger bond and a greater sense of security for both of you.

In addition to strengthening your bond with your dog, playing interactive games can also help to improve their behavior and obedience. By engaging in play with your dog, you are reinforcing positive behaviors, such as listening to commands, following cues, and respecting boundaries. Interactive games can also help to teach your dog important skills, such as impulse control, patience, and focus, which can be beneficial in other areas of their training and daily life.

Overall, creating a playful bond with your dog through interactive games is a wonderful way to show your love and affection for your furry friend. By incorporating games into your daily routine, you can provide your dog with mental stimulation, physical exercise, and a sense of connection that will strengthen your relationship and bring you closer together. So grab a toy, get outside, and start playing with your dog today!

Chapter 7: Communicating Effectively with Your Deaf or Blind Dog

Using Visual and Tactile Signals to Communicate with Deaf Dogs

Communication is key in any relationship, including the one you have with your furry companion. For dog owners with deaf dogs, finding alternative ways to communicate is essential. Using visual and tactile signals can be incredibly effective in getting your message across to your deaf dog. By incorporating these methods into your training and daily interactions, you can strengthen your bond and ensure a happy and healthy relationship with your four-legged friend.

Visual signals are a great way to communicate with deaf dogs. Hand signals can be used to give commands such as sit, stay, or come. Consistency is key when using visual signals, as your dog will learn to associate the hand movements with specific actions over time. It's important to keep these signals simple and clear to avoid confusion. For example, a closed fist may mean sit, while an open palm may mean stay. By using these visual cues consistently, you can effectively communicate with your deaf dog and reinforce positive behaviors.

Tactile signals, or physical touch, can also be a powerful way to communicate with deaf dogs. A gentle touch on the shoulder or back can signal approval or praise, while a firmer touch may indicate correction or redirection. Tactile signals can be especially useful in training, as they provide immediate feedback for your dog. By combining visual and tactile signals, you can create a comprehensive communication system that allows you to effectively convey your messages to your deaf dog.

In addition to visual and tactile signals, using other sensory cues can also help you communicate with your deaf dog. For example, you can use scent cues by using a specific fragrance or essential oil to signal certain commands or actions. You can also incorporate toys or treats as rewards for desired behaviors, further reinforcing your communication and strengthening your bond with your deaf dog. By being creative and open to different communication methods, you can find what works best for you and your furry friend.

Overall, using visual and tactile signals to communicate with deaf dogs can be a rewarding experience for both you and your pet. By being patient, consistent, and understanding, you can effectively communicate with your deaf dog and build a strong, loving relationship. Remember that each dog is unique, so it may take time to find what works best for your furry friend. With dedication and love, you can create a happy and fulfilling life with your deaf dog.

Utilizing Scent and Touch to Communicate with Blind Dogs

Blind dogs may face unique challenges when it comes to communication, but there are ways to effectively connect with them using their other senses, such as scent and touch. By utilizing these senses, you can create a stronger bond with your blind canine companion and ensure they feel loved and understood.

One way to communicate with a blind dog is through scent. Dogs have an incredible sense of smell, and they can use this to navigate their surroundings and understand their environment. You can use scents to help your blind dog identify different objects or areas in your home. For example, you can use essential oils or scent markers to indicate certain areas, such as their bed or food bowl. This can help your dog feel more secure and confident in their surroundings.

Touch is another important way to communicate with a blind dog. Physical touch can provide comfort and reassurance to your dog, helping them feel safe and loved. You can use gentle petting or massage to communicate affection and establish a strong bond with your blind dog. Additionally, you can use tactile cues, such as tapping their paw or shoulder, to indicate commands or directions. This can help your dog understand what you are asking of them and feel more connected to you.

Incorporating scent and touch into your communication with a blind dog can help strengthen your relationship and build trust. By using these senses, you can provide your dog with the guidance and support they need to navigate their world confidently. Remember to be patient and understanding with your blind dog, as they may need extra time to learn and adjust to these new forms of communication.

Overall, utilizing scent and touch to communicate with a blind dog can help you create a loving and fulfilling relationship with your canine companion. By being mindful of their unique needs and preferences, you can ensure that your blind dog feels happy, safe, and loved in your care. So take the time to explore these sensory communication methods and watch as your bond with your blind dog grows stronger each day.

Building a Strong Connection with Dogs with Hearing or Vision Impairments

Building a strong connection with dogs who have hearing or vision impairments requires a unique approach that focuses on understanding and effective communication. Dogs rely heavily on their senses of hearing and sight to navigate the world around them, so it is important to be patient and compassionate when working with them. By building a strong bond with your dog, you can help them feel safe, loved, and secure in their environment.

One of the key ways to connect with a dog who has hearing or vision impairments is through touch. Physical contact can help to reassure your dog and strengthen your bond with them. Gently petting and stroking your dog can provide them with comfort and help them feel connected to you. It is important to be sensitive to your dog's body language and cues, as they may communicate in different ways than a dog with full sensory abilities.

Another important aspect of building a strong connection with a dog who has hearing or vision impairments is through training. Training can help to establish a routine and create a sense of predictability for your dog. Using positive reinforcement techniques, such as treats and praise, can help your dog learn new commands and behaviors. It is important to be patient and consistent with your training, as it may take longer for a dog with impairments to learn new skills.

Communication is key when building a strong connection with a dog who has hearing or vision impairments. Dogs rely on cues and signals to understand their environment, so it is important to use clear and consistent communication methods. For a dog with hearing impairments, you can use hand signals or visual cues to communicate commands. For a dog with vision impairments, you can use verbal cues and physical touch to guide them. It is important to be patient and understanding when communicating with your dog, as they may require more time to respond.

Overall, building a strong connection with a dog who has hearing or vision impairments requires patience, understanding, and compassion. By focusing on touch, training, and effective communication, you can help your dog feel loved, safe, and secure in their environment. Remember to be patient and consistent in your interactions with your dog, and always prioritize their well-being and comfort. With time and effort, you can create a strong and lasting bond with your furry companion, regardless of their sensory abilities.

Chapter 8: Showing Love to Your Dog with Special Dietary Needs

Understanding Your Dog's Dietary Requirements

Proper nutrition is essential for the overall health and well-being of your furry friend. Just like humans, dogs have specific dietary requirements that need to be met in order for them to thrive. As a responsible dog owner, it is important to understand what your dog needs in terms of nutrition to ensure they lead a happy and healthy life.

Dogs require a balanced diet that includes proteins, carbohydrates, fats, vitamins, and minerals. Proteins are essential for building and repairing tissues, while carbohydrates provide energy. Fats are important for maintaining healthy skin and coat, and vitamins and minerals play a crucial role in supporting various bodily functions. It is important to choose a high-quality dog food that meets these nutritional requirements.

In addition to choosing the right dog food, it is also important to consider your dog's age, size, and activity level when determining their dietary needs. Puppies, adult dogs, and senior dogs have different nutritional requirements, so it is important to select a diet that is appropriate for your dog's life stage. Similarly, active dogs may require more calories than sedentary dogs to maintain their energy levels.

It is also important to monitor your dog's weight and adjust their diet accordingly. Obesity is a common problem among dogs and can lead to a variety of health issues. If your dog is overweight, it is important to work with your veterinarian to develop a weight loss plan that includes a balanced diet and regular exercise.

By understanding your dog's dietary requirements and providing them with a balanced diet, you can help ensure that they live a long and healthy life. Remember to consult with your veterinarian if you have any questions or concerns about your dog's nutrition, as they can provide valuable guidance and recommendations to help you make informed decisions about your dog's diet.

Providing Nutritious and Delicious Meals for Dogs with Special Needs

When it comes to caring for a dog with special dietary needs, providing nutritious and delicious meals is essential. Whether your furry friend has allergies, food sensitivities, or a medical condition that requires a specific diet, it's important to ensure that they are getting the right nutrients to support their health and well-being.

One of the first steps in creating a meal plan for a dog with special dietary needs is to consult with your veterinarian. They can help you determine what foods are safe for your dog to eat and which ones to avoid. Additionally, they may recommend specific supplements or prescription diets to help meet your dog's nutritional requirements.

When selecting ingredients for your dog's meals, opt for high-quality, whole foods that are free from artificial additives and fillers. Fresh meats, vegetables, and fruits can provide essential vitamins, minerals, and antioxidants to support your dog's overall health. Be sure to avoid common allergens such as wheat, corn, and soy, and consider rotating protein sources to prevent food sensitivities from developing.

To ensure that your dog's meals are both nutritious and delicious, consider incorporating a variety of flavors and textures into their diet. Mixing in different proteins, such as chicken, beef, and fish, can help keep mealtime interesting for your pup. You can also add in healthy fats, like coconut oil or salmon oil, to help support your dog's skin and coat health.

In addition to providing balanced meals, it's important to monitor your dog's weight and overall health regularly. Adjust their portion sizes as needed to maintain a healthy body condition, and be sure to provide plenty of fresh water throughout the day. By taking a proactive approach to your dog's nutrition, you can help them thrive and live a happy, healthy life.

Consulting with a Vet to Ensure Your Dog's Dietary Needs are Met

Consulting with a vet is crucial when it comes to ensuring that your dog's dietary needs are being met. Your veterinarian is an expert in animal nutrition and can provide valuable guidance on what foods are best for your dog based on their age, breed, size, and any underlying health conditions they may have. By consulting with a vet, you can ensure that your dog is receiving the proper balance of nutrients to support their overall health and well-being.

When consulting with a vet about your dog's dietary needs, it's important to discuss any specific dietary requirements or restrictions that your dog may have. For example, if your dog has food allergies or sensitivities, your vet can recommend hypoallergenic or limited ingredient diets that can help alleviate their symptoms. Additionally, if your dog is overweight or underweight, your vet can provide guidance on how to adjust their diet to help them reach a healthy weight.

In addition to discussing your dog's specific dietary needs, your vet can also provide guidance on portion control and feeding schedules. It's important to feed your dog the appropriate amount of food based on their age, size, and activity level to prevent obesity or malnourishment. Your vet can help you determine the right portion sizes and feeding frequency for your dog to ensure they are getting the right amount of nutrition without overeating.

Consulting with a vet is also important when it comes to choosing the right type of food for your dog. Your vet can recommend high-quality commercial dog foods that meet the nutritional requirements set by the Association of American Feed Control Officials (AAFCO). They can also provide guidance on whether a raw diet, homemade diet, or specialty diet is appropriate for your dog based on their individual needs.

Overall, consulting with a vet is essential for ensuring that your dog's dietary needs are met. By working closely with your vet, you can develop a customized feeding plan that meets your dog's specific nutritional requirements and helps them maintain optimal health. Your vet is a valuable resource when it comes to providing the best care for your furry friend, so don't hesitate to reach out for guidance on your dog's diet.

Chapter 9: Creating a Safe and Comfortable Environment for Your Dog

Dog-Proofing Your Home to Keep Your Dog Safe

Ensuring the safety and well-being of your furry friend is essential as a responsible dog owner. Dog-proofing your home is a crucial step in creating a safe environment for your canine companion. By taking the necessary precautions, you can prevent accidents and keep your dog happy and healthy.

One of the first steps in dog-proofing your home is to secure any hazardous items that may be within your dog's reach. This includes household chemicals, medications, and small objects that could be swallowed. Keep these items locked away in cabinets or high shelves to prevent your dog from getting into them.

Another important aspect of dog-proofing is to secure your home's electrical cords and outlets. Dogs are curious creatures and may chew on cords or stick their noses into outlets, posing a serious risk of electrocution. Use cord protectors or hide cords behind furniture to prevent your dog from accessing them.

Additionally, it is essential to secure your trash bins to prevent your dog from rummaging through them and potentially ingesting harmful substances. Invest in a sturdy trash can with a secure lid or keep it in a cabinet to avoid any accidents.

Creating a safe space for your dog to relax and play is also important. Make sure to provide a comfortable bed, toys, and water bowls in designated areas of your home. Keep any toxic plants out of reach and consider installing baby gates to restrict access to certain areas of your home.

By taking these simple steps to dog-proof your home, you can create a safe and comfortable environment for your canine companion.

Remember, the safety and well-being of your dog should always be a top priority as a loving and responsible pet owner.

Providing a Cozy and Relaxing Space for Your Dog

Creating a cozy and relaxing space for your dog is essential in ensuring their comfort and well-being. Dogs, like humans, appreciate having a designated area where they can feel safe and secure. By providing a cozy space for your furry friend, you are showing them that you care about their happiness and overall quality of life.

When designing a cozy space for your dog, consider their specific needs and preferences. Some dogs may prefer a soft bed or blanket to curl up on, while others may enjoy a cozy dog house or crate. Make sure to place their bed or crate in a quiet and comfortable area of your home, away from any loud noises or distractions.

In addition to a comfortable bed or crate, consider adding some soothing elements to your dog's space. This could include calming essential oils, a cozy blanket with your scent on it, or a calming music playlist to help them relax. Creating a peaceful environment for your dog will not only help them feel more at ease, but it will also strengthen the bond between you and your furry companion.

It's also important to keep your dog's space clean and tidy. Regularly wash their bedding, vacuum the area, and remove any clutter that may be causing them stress. Dogs are sensitive to their environment, so keeping their space clean and organized will help them feel more relaxed and content.

By providing a cozy and relaxing space for your dog, you are not only enhancing their quality of life, but you are also strengthening your bond with them. Remember, a happy and comfortable dog is a healthy and well-loved dog. So take the time to create a space that your furry friend will truly appreciate and enjoy.

Ensuring Your Dog Feels Secure and Comfortable in Their Environment

Ensuring Your Dog Feels Secure and Comfortable in Their Environment is crucial for their overall well-being and happiness. As dog owners, it is our responsibility to create a safe and comfortable space for our furry friends to thrive. One of the first steps in achieving this is to provide a designated area for your dog that is their own. Whether it's a cozy bed, a crate, or a corner of the room, having a space that belongs solely to your dog can help them feel secure and at ease.

In addition to a designated space, it's important to establish a routine for your dog. Dogs thrive on consistency and knowing what to expect. By providing a regular schedule for feeding, playtime, walks, and bedtime, you are creating a sense of stability and security for your dog. This routine can help reduce anxiety and stress, making your dog feel more comfortable in their environment.

Another way to ensure your dog feels secure and comfortable is to provide them with plenty of mental and physical stimulation. Dogs are intelligent and active creatures that need both mental and physical exercise to stay healthy and happy. By incorporating playtime, training sessions, and interactive toys into your dog's daily routine, you are not only keeping them physically fit but also mentally stimulated and fulfilled.

Creating a safe environment for your dog is also essential in helping them feel secure and comfortable. Make sure your home is free of hazards such as toxic plants, small objects that can be swallowed, and secure any loose wires or cords that could pose a danger to your dog. Providing a comfortable temperature, access to clean water, and a comfortable bed are also important factors in creating a safe and comfortable environment for your furry friend.

By following these tips and guidelines, you can ensure that your dog feels secure and comfortable in their environment. A happy and comfortable dog is more likely to bond with you, trust you, and show you love and affection in return. Remember, your dog's well-being and happiness should always be a top priority as a responsible pet owner.

Chapter 10: Celebrating Special Occasions with Your Dog

Birthday Parties and Other Special Celebrations for Your Dog

Birthday parties and other special celebrations are a fun and exciting way to show love and appreciation for your furry friend. Just like humans, dogs love to be celebrated and pampered on their special day. Whether your dog is turning one year old or reaching a milestone age, throwing a birthday party can be a great way to bond with your pet and create lasting memories.

When planning a birthday party for your dog, consider their likes and dislikes. Think about their favorite toys, treats, and activities to incorporate into the celebration. You can also invite their furry friends to join in on the fun, creating a social and interactive environment for your pet. Don't forget to set up a special area for your dog to relax and unwind if they become overwhelmed by the excitement.

In addition to birthday parties, there are many other special occasions that you can celebrate with your dog. Whether it's National Pet Day, Halloween, or even their adoption anniversary, there are endless opportunities to show love and appreciation for your furry companion. Consider hosting a themed party or taking your dog on a special outing to mark the occasion.

Celebrating special occasions with your dog is not only a fun way to bond with your pet, but it also helps strengthen the relationship between you and your furry friend. By taking the time to plan a special celebration, you are showing your dog that they are a valued member of the family. This can help build trust and create a deeper connection between you and your pet.

Overall, birthday parties and other special celebrations are a great way to show love and appreciation for your dog. Whether it's a small gathering with family or a larger event with friends, celebrating special occasions with your furry friend is a fun and meaningful way to create lasting memories. So go ahead, plan a special celebration for your dog and watch as they enjoy being the center of attention on their special day.

Including Your Dog in Holiday Festivities

The holidays are a time for celebration, and what better way to spread the joy than by including your furry friend in the festivities? Dogs are members of the family, so it's only natural to want to involve them in the holiday fun. Whether you're hosting a gathering at home or attending a holiday party elsewhere, there are plenty of ways to include your dog in the merriment.

One way to include your dog in holiday festivities is by dressing them up in festive attire. Whether it's a Santa hat, reindeer antlers, or a cozy holiday sweater, dressing your dog in seasonal gear can add an extra element of fun to the celebrations. Just be sure to choose outfits that are comfortable for your dog and allow them to move freely.

Another way to involve your dog in holiday festivities is by including them in holiday photos. Whether you're sending out holiday cards or simply capturing memories for yourself, having your dog in the picture can make the moment even more special. Consider setting up a festive backdrop or props to make the photos even more festive.

When it comes to holiday meals, it's important to remember that many traditional holiday foods can be harmful to dogs. While it's okay to treat your dog to a special holiday meal, be sure to stick to dog-friendly ingredients and avoid foods that are toxic to dogs, such as chocolate, grapes, and onions. You can also consider making homemade dog treats to share with your furry friend during the holiday season.

In addition to dressing up, taking photos, and enjoying special holiday treats, there are plenty of other ways to include your dog in holiday festivities. Consider taking your dog on a holiday-themed walk or hike, attending a pet-friendly holiday event, or even hosting a dog-friendly holiday party of your own. Whatever you choose to do, involving your dog in holiday festivities is a great way to show them love and make lasting memories together.

Creating Lasting Memories with Your Dog on Special Occasions

Creating lasting memories with your dog on special occasions is a wonderful way to strengthen your bond and show your love for your furry friend. Whether it's celebrating their birthday, adoption anniversary, or just a random day dedicated to them, there are many ways to make these moments special and memorable.

One way to create lasting memories with your dog on special occasions is to plan a fun outing or adventure together. Take your dog to their favorite park, beach, or hiking trail for a day of exploration and quality time together. You can also plan a special picnic or outdoor meal with your dog, complete with their favorite treats and toys.

Another way to create lasting memories with your dog on special occasions is to involve them in the celebration. For example, you can bake a dog-friendly cake or treat for their birthday, or create a special photo shoot to capture the moment. Including your dog in the festivities will make them feel loved and appreciated.

In addition to outings and celebrations, you can also create lasting memories with your dog through training and play. Teach your dog a new trick or skill, play their favorite games, or simply spend time cuddling and relaxing together. These moments of connection and bonding will create lasting memories that you both will cherish.

Overall, creating lasting memories with your dog on special occasions is all about showing your love and appreciation for your furry friend. Whether it's a simple gesture or a grand celebration, the important thing is to make your dog feel special and loved. These moments will not only strengthen your bond, but also create memories that will last a lifetime.

Chapter 11: Coping with the Loss of a Beloved Pet

Grieving the Loss of Your Dog

Losing a beloved pet can be one of the most difficult experiences a pet owner can go through. The loss of a dog, who is often considered a member of the family, can be particularly devastating. Grieving the loss of your dog is a process that takes time and patience, and it is important to allow yourself to feel and process your emotions during this difficult time.

It is normal to feel a range of emotions when grieving the loss of your dog, including sadness, anger, guilt, and even denial. Allow yourself to feel these emotions and don't be afraid to seek support from friends, family, or a therapist who can help you navigate through your grief. Remember that it is okay to grieve in your own way and at your own pace.

One way to cope with the loss of your dog is to create a special memorial in honor of your furry friend. This can be as simple as a photo collage or as elaborate as planting a tree in their memory. Finding a way to honor your dog's memory can bring comfort and closure during the grieving process.

Another helpful way to cope with the loss of your dog is to talk about your feelings and memories with others who loved your dog. Sharing stories and memories can help you process your grief and celebrate the life of your beloved pet. Consider creating a scrapbook or memory box filled with photos, toys, and other mementos that remind you of your dog.

Remember that it is important to take care of yourself during this difficult time. Make sure to eat well, get plenty of rest, and engage in activities that bring you joy and comfort. It is also important to give yourself time to heal and to be gentle with yourself as you navigate through the grieving process. By allowing yourself to grieve and honoring the memory of your dog, you can eventually find peace and healing in your heart.

Honoring Your Dog's Memory

Losing a beloved pet can be one of the most difficult experiences a dog owner may face. The bond we share with our furry friends is incredibly special, and their passing can leave a void in our hearts. It is important to honor and remember our dogs in a meaningful way, as they have brought so much love and joy into our lives.

One way to honor your dog's memory is by creating a memorial in their honor. This can be a physical memorial such as a plaque or headstone in your yard, or a digital memorial on social media or a pet memorial website. You can also create a memory box filled with your dog's favorite toys, photos, and other mementos that remind you of them.

Another way to honor your dog's memory is by giving back to other animals in need. Consider making a donation to a local animal shelter or rescue organization in your dog's name, or volunteer your time to help animals in need. This is a beautiful way to pay tribute to your dog's legacy and continue their spirit of love and compassion.

It is also important to take care of yourself during this difficult time. Grieving the loss of a pet is a natural process, and it is okay to feel sadness, anger, and other emotions. Reach out to friends, family, or a support group for comfort and understanding, and give yourself permission to mourn your beloved dog in your own way.

Lastly, remember that your dog's memory will always live on in your heart. Cherish the special moments you shared together, and know that your dog's love will never truly be gone. By honoring your dog's memory in a meaningful way, you can keep their spirit alive and continue to feel their presence in your life.

Finding Comfort and Support in the Aftermath of Losing a Pet

Losing a beloved pet can be one of the most heartbreaking experiences a dog owner can face. The grief and sadness that accompany the loss of a furry companion can feel overwhelming, leaving many pet owners feeling lost and alone. In the aftermath of losing a pet, it is important to find comfort and support to help navigate through the difficult emotions that come with saying goodbye.

One way to find comfort and support in the aftermath of losing a pet is to lean on friends and family members who understand the deep bond between a pet and their owner. Surrounding yourself with loved ones who can offer a listening ear and a shoulder to cry on can provide much-needed emotional support during this challenging time. Sharing memories and stories about your pet with others who loved them can also help in the healing process.

Another way to find comfort and support after losing a pet is to seek out support groups or online communities of fellow pet owners who have also experienced loss. Connecting with others who are going through similar emotions can provide a sense of validation and understanding that can be comforting during a time of grief. These support groups can offer a safe space to share feelings, seek guidance, and find solace in the shared love for animals.

Engaging in self-care practices can also be beneficial in finding comfort and support after losing a pet. Taking time to prioritize your own emotional well-being through activities such as meditation, journaling, or spending time in nature can help in processing grief and finding moments of peace and tranquility. It is important to be gentle with yourself during this time and allow yourself to grieve in whatever way feels most natural to you.

Lastly, finding ways to honor the memory of your beloved pet can bring comfort and support in the aftermath of their passing. Creating a memorial, planting a tree, or making a donation to a pet charity in your pet's name are all meaningful ways to pay tribute to the love and joy they brought into your life. Finding ways to keep their memory alive can bring a sense of comfort and closure as you navigate through the grieving process. Remember, it is okay to seek help and support during this difficult time, and know that you are not alone in your sorrow.

www.ingramcontent.com/pod-product-compliance
Lightning Source LLC
Chambersburg PA
CBHW050706250726

48662CB00002B/880